FIXING OBESITY

HOW TO OVERCOME FOOD CRAVING, LOSE WEIGHT, AND BOOST YOUR ENERGY.

BY

MARK K. BENTON

TABLE OF CONTENTS

Obesity is a complicated, multifaceted disease. The cause is accumulated excess body fat. A person is considered obese if their body mass index (BMI, kg/m2) is greater than or equal to 30, whereas being overweight is defined as having a BMI between 25 and 29.9. An unparalleled epidemic of obesity is growing faster and faster. Throughout the past 50 years, there has been a noticeable rise in obesity rates globally.

An increased body mass index (BMI) increases the risk of developing non-communicable diseases like diabetes, cardiovascular disease, and musculoskeletal disorders, which dramatically reduces life expectancy and quality of life. Long-term energy imbalance between calories ingested and calories burned is the primary factor causing obesity.

According to recommendations from the World Health Organization (WHO), BMI is used to define and diagnose obesity.

In addition, there are three severity categories for obesity: class I (BMI 30.0–34.9), class II (BMI 35.0–39.9), and class III (BMI 40.0).

All age groups and genders now experience significantly greater rates of obesity, with older people and women seeing proportionately higher prevalence rates.

Food Consumption and Unbalanced Energy

The primary reasons for obesity are still somewhat debatable. Increased energy from more readily available, highly satisfying, and energy-dense foods that are heavy in fat and carbohydrates has contributed significantly to the obesity pandemic. Diet and other social, economic, and environmental aspects of the food supply all have an impact on how well a person can maintain balance. In a 13-year follow-up study involving 3,000 young people, it was discovered that those who consumed significantly more fast food weighed an average of 6 kg more and had bigger waist circumferences than those who consumed the least. They were also discovered to have greater rates of harmful weight-related health problems, such as excessive triglyceride levels and a twofold increased risk of getting MetS. These problems are even worse in some people who have a genetic sensitivity to fat accumulation.

The predisposition for obesity is influenced by psychological, lifestyle, and family history variables. The risk of obesity can be increased by family genetics (propensity to collect fat) or lifestyle factors, as well as by nature and nurture (poor dietary or exercise habits). A child who has one fat parent has a three-fold increased risk of being obese as an adult, while a child who has two obese parents has a ten-fold increased risk. A cross-sectional observational study of 260 kids (139 girls and 121 boys, 2.4 to 17.2 years old) found that obesity and cardio metabolic disease history in the family are major risk factors for the severity of childhood obesity.

The body receives instructions from the genes on how to react to changes in its surroundings. Studies of similarities and variances among relatives, twins, and adoptees provide indirect scientific proof that genetic variables account for a large amount of the diversity in adult weight.

Genes can induce obesity in a variety of ways, generically categorized as:

Monogenic cause

The leptin-melanocortin pathway is the main location of monogenic causes, which are those brought on by a single gene mutation.

Syndromic obesity

Obesity with other phenotypes, such as neurodevelopmental disorders and another organ/system malformations, is referred to as syndromic obesity.

Polygenic obesity

A significant number of genes collectively contribute to polygenic obesity, which is exacerbated by an environment that "promotes weight gain."

Hormones have a factor in obesity and overweight, in addition to increasing consumption of foods high in energy and genes.

The endocrine system, a network of glands, secretes hormones into our bloodstream. To help our body handle various situations and challenges, the endocrine system collaborates with the neurological system and the immune system. Obesity can result from hormonal excesses or deficiencies, and vice versa; obesity can result from hormonal alterations.

Leptin, insulin, sex hormones, growth hormone, and others have all been thoroughly investigated for their function in obesity and an increase in body weight. These hormones affect hunger, metabolism, body fat distribution, and the enhanced storage of extra calories as fats in the diet.

The following hormones are some of those crucial to the pathology of obesity:

Adipocytes produce the hormone leptin, which is then released into the bloodstream. By exerting its effects on particular brain regions, leptin lessens a person's desire to eat. It also appears to have a say in how the body handles its fat reserves.

Leptin is created by fat, hence individuals who are obese typically have higher leptin levels than those who are of normal weight. However, despite having higher amounts of this hormone that suppresses hunger, obese persons are less sensitive to its effects and, as a result, tend not to experience satiety during and after meals.

Insulin boosts the blood's supply of glucose (sugar) to tissues like muscles, the liver, and fat. This procedure is crucial to maintaining appropriate levels of blood glucose and ensuring that there is energy available for daily activities.

When insulin signals are lost in an obese person, tissues lose their ability to regulate sugar (glucose) levels.

The distribution of body fat has a significant impact on the emergence of obesity-related diseases such as heart disease, stroke, and various types of arthritis. A larger risk of disease is associated with abdominal fat than with fat that is stored on the hips, thighs, or bottom. The distribution of body fat is influenced by androgens (in men) and estrogens (in females).

The testicles and ovaries of males and postmenopausal women do not produce a lot of estrogens. However, compared to what is produced in the ovaries, the majority of their estrogen is created in body fat.

Androgen production in the testes is high in younger males. These levels gradually decline as the man ages.

Variations in body fat distribution are related to changes in sex hormone levels with aging in both men and women. Older males and postmenopausal women tend to increase the accumulation of fat around their belly (making them "apple-shaped"), whilst women of childbearing age tend to store fat in their lower body (making them "pear-shaped"). Women who are postmenopausal and taking estrogen pills do not develop belly fat.

Growth hormone

Growth hormone is produced by the pituitary gland in our brain, which affects a person's height and promotes the development of bone and muscle. Growth hormone influences metabolism as well (the rate at which we burn kilojoules for energy). Growth hormone levels have been discovered to be lower in obese individuals than in individuals of normal weight.

The body can be retrained to burn excess body fat and keep it off through long-term behavior adjustments like healthy eating and frequent exercise. Studies have also indicated that losing weight with a balanced diet, regular exercise, or bariatric surgery improves insulin sensitivity, reduces inflammation, and has a positive impact on the hormones associated with obesity. Losing weight is also linked to a lower risk of heart disease, stroke, type II diabetes, and several types of cancer.

HOW ADDED SUGAR AFFECT WEIGHT GAIN.

A diet high in added sugars is a contributing factor in weight gain and chronic illnesses like diabetes, heart disease, and obesity

The complicated and multifaceted processes by which consuming added sugar contributes to weight gain and an increase in body fat are discussed.

Here are effects of added sugar on weight gain.

Added sugar has little to no nutritional benefits and is a source of empty calories. Foods with a lot of added sugar have a high-calorie content, which leads to weight gain.

High-sugar diets cause long-lasting blood sugar elevations, insulin resistance, and leptin resistance, all of which are connected to weight gain and excess body fat.

Protein and fiber, which are vital nutrients for helping you feel full and satisfied, are typically lacking in high-sugar foods and beverages.

Added sugars replace nutritious foods, can cause weight gain, and raise your chance of developing chronic illnesses like heart disease.

Your brain's reward regions and hormones that control your appetite are both impacted by sugar, which may make you want more delicious meals and lead to overeating.

Overindulging in added sugar can result in weight gain and greatly raise your risk of developing chronic illnesses including diabetes, heart disease, and obesity.

Unsaturated fats

Unsaturated fats, are regarded as healthy fats because they have a range of positive effects on health. These effects are lower blood cholesterol levels, less inflammation, and stable cardiac rhythms. Vegetable oils and seeds are examples of foods that are high in unsaturated fats.

Two categories of "healthy" unsaturated fats exist:

1. Monounsaturated fats can be found in:

Canola, peanut, and olive oils

Avocados

nuts like pecans, hazelnuts, and almonds

pumpkin with sesame seeds, for example

2. There are polyunsaturated fats in:

oils from flaxseed, corn, soybeans, and sunflower

Walnuts

hemp seeds

Fish

Olive oil - It is a good source of polyunsaturated fat while having a larger concentration of monounsaturated fat.

omega-3 fat is an essential kind of polyunsaturated fat (it cannot be produced by the body), required from food. E.g fish, walnuts, canola or soya bean oil , and flax seed.

Saturated fat is found in healthful foods. Although plant foods like coconut and palm fruit are high in saturated fats, saturated fat is mostly found in animal meals.

A diet high in saturated fats can raise your total cholesterol and shift the ratio in favor of more dangerous LDL cholesterol, which increases your risk of artery blockages in your heart and other organs. Your risk of heart disease is increased by LDL cholesterol. Saturated fat is also known as unhealthy fats.

Saturated fat can be found in food like:

 beef, lamb, and pork

Chicken and other poultry

dairy goods made with whole milk, such as milk, cheese, and ice cream

Butter\sEggs

Coconut and palm oil

Here are several weight-loss strategies that emphasize careful carbohydrate selection and healthy eating, which help to decrease your hunger and desire while keeping you full and leading to sustained weight loss over time. And assist in enhancing your metabolic health.

Rapid weight loss is rarely long-lasting, but when you concentrate on long-term health and behaviors you can maintain, it will help you improve your health and increase the likelihood that you will lose weight.

1. Reducing refined carbs

Reducing your intake of carbohydrates can help you lose weight quickly. This could be accomplished by following a diet that is low in carbohydrates. Also by consuming less processed carbohydrates and more whole grains.

If that is achieved, your hunger decreases , and you often consume fewer calories as a result. With a diet that has low carbohydrate levels, you will use your body's fat reserves as energy instead of carbohydrates. It benefits to increase fiber intake (slows digestion) and more complex carbohydrates, such as whole grains, coupled with a calorie deficit. A low-carbohydrate diet might be challenging to follow, resulting in less success in maintaining a healthy weight. Reduced-calorie diets are simple to follow for long periods of time and can also result in weight loss.

Reducing refined carbohydrates may reduce insulin levels, make you feel fuller for longer, and aid in weight loss.

2. Consume vegetables, fat, and protein.

Your meals should contain the following :

 protein, fat, vegetables and whole grains.

Protein

When trying to lose weight, it's crucial to consume the right quantity of protein to maintain your health and muscle mass.

The average male needs 56–91 grams of protein daily and the average female 46–75 grams.

Suitable sources of protein include:

Meat: lamb, hog, chicken, and beef

Salmon, trout, sardines, shrimp eggs, and other fish and seafood

Vegetable proteins (beans, lentils, quinoa, tempeh, and tofu).

Vegetables

Vegetables are nutrient-rich, and you can consume a lot of them without significantly raising your calorie and carbohydrate intake.

All vegetables are enriched with nutrient and beneficial additions to your diet, but some, (corn, potatoes, and sweet potatoes) have greater carbohydrate levels, due to high fiber content. These vegetables are complex carbohydrates.

Vegetables to increase intake of are:

broccoli

cauliflower\spinach\tomatoes

kale

Belgian spuds

cabbage

Geneva chard

lettuce

cucumber\peppers

Wholesome fats

Don't be hesitant to eat fats.

Healthy fat is needed in any diet you adopt. You should definitely include avocados, nuts, seeds, olives, and olive oil in your diet. They are nutritious additions.

Due to their higher saturated fat content, other fats like butter and coconut oil should only be used seldom.

Leafy greens are a great source of nutrients, low in calories, and a great way to bulk up a meal.

Increasing your water intake is a simple strategy to support weight loss with little effort. A study found that after 30–40 minutes, consuming 16.9 ounces (500 ml) of water temporarily boosted the number of calories burnt by 30%. Consuming water prior to a meal speed up weight reduction and cut calories.

These meal plan are examples of low carbohydrate diet plan. A source of Protein, healthy fats, and vegetables should be found in every meal. Everyone has varied demands and culinary preferences. Therefore these are options you can pick from.

Idea for breakfast

1. poached egg, sliced avocado, and berries on the side.

2. Quiche without a crust, with spinach, mushrooms, and feta.

3. A-side of cottage cheese unsweetened Greek yogurt with berries and nuts and a green smoothie made with spinach, avocado, and nut milk are also served.

Ideas for lunch

1. grilled chicken, black beans, red pepper, and salsa in a lettuce wrap with smoked salmon, avocado, and a side of asparagus.

2. BLT wrap with celery sticks and peanut butter, a kale and spinach salad with grilled tofu, chickpeas, and guacamole

Ideas for dinner

1. Chicken, peppers, mango, avocado, and spices in an enchilada salad

2. a baked turkey dish with cheese, peppers, onions, and mushrooms

3. Roasted cauliflower with tempeh, Brussels sprouts, and pine nuts is part of an antipasto salad that includes white beans, asparagus, cucumbers, olive oil, and Parmesan.

4. Salmon baked with roasted zucchini, ginger, and sesame oil

Snack ideas

1. Broccoli, hummus, and vegetables

2. Homemade trail mix made with nuts and dried fruit is healthful.

3. Flaxseeds with cinnamon in cottage cheese

4. Roast chickpeas with a kick

5. Roasted seeds from a pumpkin

6. Edamame and steamed tuna pouches.

1. Opt for diet-friendly foods.

Choose food that are healthy and preferable for losing weight.

2. Consume more fiber.

Increasing your fiber intake is a systematic weight loss approach that can help decrease stomach emptying and keep you feeling fuller for longer. Whole grains, fruits, vegetables, nuts, seeds, and other high-fiber foods contain fiber.

3. Take tea or coffee.

Consuming caffeine may speed up your metabolism. However, you should take care not to consume much added sugars in these beverages.

4. Make whole foods the foundation of your diet. They are enrich with nutrient, satisfying, and prevent overeating.

5. Eat slowly.

Eating slowly makes you feel more satisfied and increases the production of hormones that help you lose weight while eating fastly will result to overweight. (over time)

6. Get a decent night's rest.

Poor sleep is a major risk factors for weight gain, which is one of the many reasons why proper sleep is crucial if one is to lose weight.

7. Limit fruit juice and beverages with added sugar. Sugar contains high calorie that prevent weight loss.

8. Make an energy deficit

To reduce weight, you should eat less than your body daily need. The higher the calorie deficit you have determines how quickly you lose weight.

For instance, losing more weight than eating 200 fewer calories each day is likely to require 500 fewer calories each for eight weeks.

9. Move your body

Exercise aid weight loss process. Weightlifting, in particular, has many advantages.

You'll burn calories while lifting weights, preventing your metabolism from slowing down, which is a common symptom of weight loss. Exercise that boosts your heart rate, or aerobic exercise, or cardio, helps you lose weight and improves your overall health by causing your body to burn more calories. Examples of cardio exercises include walking, jogging, running, cycling, and swimming.

Weightlifting is a training that is excellent for losing weight. Exercises that involve cardio are also helpful if that is not possible.

10. Eat more wisely

To reduce hunger between meals, choosing healthy low-calorie snacks is a fantastic way to lose weight.

Pick protein, vegetables and fiber-rich foods to help you feel full.

11. Maintain Control Over Stress

Long-term weight gain is aided when stress levels are higher.

Additionally, stress has been linked to overeating through changing eating habits.

12. Use small pates

By using a smaller plate to serve your meal, you encourage portion management and accelerate weight loss.

One study revealed that individuals who used a smaller plate ate less and were more pleased than those who used a normal-sized plate, despite the fact that evidence is still few and inconsistent.

13. Take a supplement with probiotics

Probiotics are microorganisms that can be taken as dietary supplements to enhance gut health.

Probiotics can aid in weight loss by boosting fat depletion and modifying hormone levels to control appetite.

14. Have a wholesome breakfast.

Eating a healthy breakfast and at a regular time can give you a head start on the day and keep you satisfied until your next meal.

15. Test Out Intermittent Fasting

Intermittent fasting is a process that involves alternating between eating and not eating in a period of time. Fasting intervals are usually between 14 and 24 hours, Intermittent fasting is beneficial as reducing calories when it comes to weight loss.

16. Reducing added sugar

Added sugar is vital in gaining weight and catastrophic medical conditions like diabetes and heart disease.

Foods containing a lot of added sugar are rich in calorie but deficient in the vitamins, minerals, fiber, and protein your body needs to function properly.

Conclusion

Although weight loss may be more rapid at the beginning of a program, experts advise losing 1% of your body weight, or roughly 1-3 pounds (0.45-1.36 kg), weekly.

Remember that you might lose more some weeks while losing less or nothing at all other others.